Keto Chaffle Recipes Cookbook

Tasty and Healthy Recipes to do at Home with your Waffle Maker

Reyhan Hoque

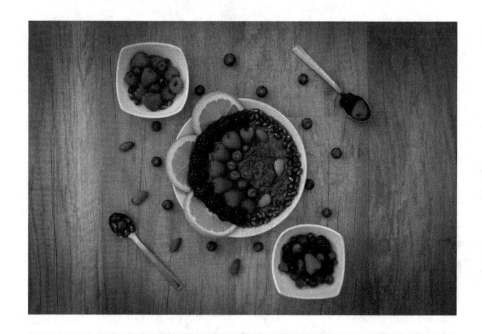

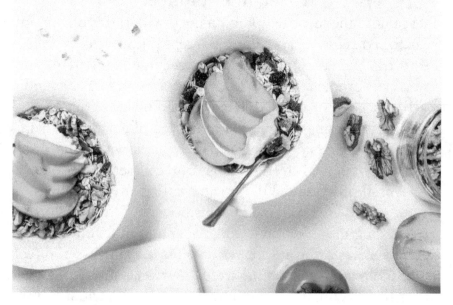

TABLE OF CONTENTS

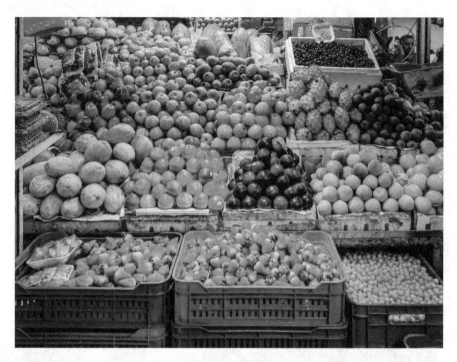

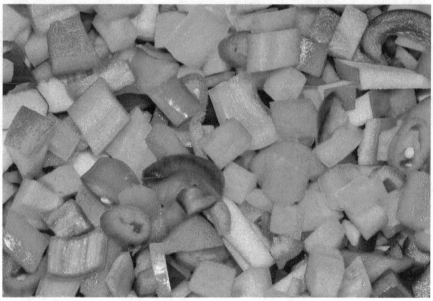

INTRODUCTION

A chaffle, or cheese waffle, is an egg and cheese keto waffle. Chaffles become a popular snack of keto / low-carb. Chaffle is made with coconut and pumpkin, making it a healthy low-carb alternative for anyone looking to lose weight. The chaffle helps stabilize blood sugar levels so the body has an easier time sensing when food is needed. The keto chaffle contains no calories or carbs, making it an ideal tool for anyone looking to lose or maintain their weight.

What is this keto Chaffle recipe in the world that has overtaken and conquered the keto community? Simply put, it's a cheese and egg waffle. There have been various variants in Facebook groups since the original recipe came out

How to make crispy chaffle

First off, beat one egg in a mixing bowl until you achieve the desired consistency and add ½ cup of finely shredded mozzarella cheese. Preheat the mini waffle iron then pour the mixture into it

If you find the taste too eggy, you can add a tablespoon of almond flour or any keto-friendly flour like coconut flour, psyllium husk flour, ground flax seed and the like. You can also top it with sugar free syrup and butter.

You can also try other kinds of cheese to see what will make your taste buds happier.

If you want it crunchier, you have to sprinkle shredded cheese on the waffle maker first and let it melt for half a minute before adding the mixture.

This is just the classic chaffle though. Remember that you can be creative with it and possibilities are endless!

Chaffles can be used for hamburger bun, hotdog bun, sandwich and pizza crust. You can also make it sweet or savory.

11 Tips to Make Chaffles

- **Preheat Well:** Yes! It sounds obvious to preheat the waffle iron before usage. However, preheating the iron moderately will not get your chaffles as crispy as you will like. The best way to preheat before cooking is to ensure that the iron is very hot.

- **Not-So-Cheesy:** Will you prefer to have your chaffles less cheesy? Then, use mozzarella cheese.
- **Not-So Eggy**: If you aren't comfortable with the smell of eggs in your chaffles, try using egg whites instead of egg yolks or whole eggs.
- **To Shred or to Slice:** Many recipes call for shredded cheese when making chaffles, but I find sliced cheeses to offer crispier pieces. While I stick with mostly shredded cheese for convenience's sake, be at ease to use sliced cheese in the same quantity. When using sliced cheeses, arrange two to four pieces in the waffle iron, top with the beaten eggs, and some slices of the cheese. Cover and cook until crispy.
- **Shallower Irons:** For better crisps on your chaffles, use shallower waffle irons as they cook easier and faster.
- **Layering:** Don't fill up the waffle iron with too much batter. Work between a quarter and a half cup of total ingredients per batch for correctly done chaffles.
- **Patience:** It is a virtue even when making chaffles. For the best results, allow the chaffles to sit in the iron for 5 to 7 minutes before serving.
- **No Peeking:** 7 minutes isn't too much of a time to wait for the outcome of your chaffles, in my opinion. Opening the iron and checking on the chaffle before it is done stands you a worse chance of ruining it.
- **Crispy Cooling:** For better crisp, I find that allowing the chaffles to cool further after they are transferred to a plate aids a lot.
- **Easy Cleaning:** For the best cleanup, wet a paper towel and wipe the inner parts of the iron clean while still warm. Kindly note that the iron should be warm but not hot!
- **Brush It:** Also, use a clean toothbrush to clean between the iron's teeth for a thorough cleanup. You may also use a dry, rough sponge to clean the iron while it is still warm

CHAPTER 1:

BREAKFAST CHAFFLE

RECIPES

1. Blueberry Shortcake Chaffles

Difficulty level: Easy

Preparation time: 10 minutes

Cooking time: 14 minutes

Servings: 2

Ingredients:

- 1 egg, beaten

- 1 tbsp cream cheese, softened

- ¼ cup finely grated mozzarella cheese

- 1/4 tsp baking powder

- 4 fresh blueberries

- 1 tsp blueberry extract

Directions:

1. Preheat the waffle iron.

2. In a medium bowl, mix all the ingredients.

3. Open the iron, pour in half of the batter, close, and cook until crispy, 6 to 7 minutes.

4. Remove the chaffle onto a plate and set aside.

5. Make the other chaffle with the remaining batter.

6. Allow cooling and enjoy after.

Nutrition: Calories: 99 Cal Total Fat: 8 g Saturated Fat: 0 g Cholesterol: 0 mg Sodium: 0 mg Carbs: 4 g

2. Crab Chaffles

Difficulty level: Medium **Preparation Time:** 10 minutes

Cooking Time: 25 minutes

Servings: 6

Ingredients:

- 1 lb crab meat

- 1/3 cup Panko breadcrumbs

- One egg

- 2 tbsp fat Greek yoghurt

- 1 tsp Dijon mustard

- 2 tbsp parsley and chives, fresh

- 1 tsp Italian seasoning

- One lemon, juiced

- Salt, pepper to taste

Directions:

1. Preheat, the waffle maker

2. Mix all the ingredients in a small mixing bowl, except crab meat.

3. Add the meat. Mix well.

4. Form the mixture into round patties.

5. Cook 1 patty for 3 minutes

6. Remove it and repeat the process with the remaining crab chaffle mixture.

7. Once ready, remove and enjoy warm.

Nutrition: Calories: 99 Cal Total Fat: 8 g Saturated Fat: 0 g Cholesterol: 0 mg Sodium: 0 mg Total Carbs: 4 g Fibre: 0 g Sugar: 0 g Protein: 16 g

3. <u>Raspberry-Pecan Chaffles</u>

Difficulty level: Medium

Preparation time: 10 minutes

Cooking time: 14 minutes

Servings: 2

Ingredients:

- 1 egg, beaten

- ½ cup finely grated mozzarella cheese

- 1 tbsp cream cheese, softened

- 1 tbsp sugar-free maple syrup

- ¼ tsp raspberry extract

- ¼ tsp vanilla extract

- 2 tbsp sugar-free caramel sauce for topping

- 3 tbsp chopped pecans for topping

Directions:

1. Preheat the waffle iron.

2. In a medium bowl, mix all the ingredients.

3. Open the iron, pour in half of the batter, close, and cook until crispy, 6 to 7 minutes.

4. Remove the chaffle onto a plate and set aside.

5. Make another chaffle with the remaining batter.

6. To serve: drizzle the caramel sauce on the chaffles and top with the pecans.

Nutrition: Calories: 99 Cal Total Fat: 8 g Saturated Fat: 0 g Cholesterol: 0 mg Sodium: 0 mg Total Carbs: 3 g

4. <u>Mixed Berry-Vanilla Chaffles</u>

Difficulty level: Medium **Preparation time:** 10 minutes

Cooking time: 28 minutes

Servings: 4

Ingredients:

- 1 egg, beaten

- ½ cup finely grated mozzarella cheese

- 1 tbsp cream cheese, softened

- 1 tbsp sugar-free maple syrup

- 2 strawberries, sliced

- 2 raspberries, slices

- ¼ tsp blackberry extract

- ¼ tsp vanilla extract

- ½ cup plain yogurt for serving

Directions:

1. Preheat the waffle iron.

2. In a medium bowl, mix all the ingredients except the yogurt.

3. Open the iron, lightly grease with cooking spray and pour in a quarter of the mixture.

4. Close the iron and cook until golden brown and crispy, 7 minutes.

5. Remove the chaffle onto a plate and set aside.

6. Make three more chaffles with the remaining mixture.

7. To serve: top with the yogurt and enjoy.

Nutrition: Calories: 99 Cal Total Fat: 8 g Saturated Fat: 0 g Cholesterol: 0 mg Sodium: 0 mg Total Carbs: 4 g

5. Ham And Cheddar Chaffles

Difficulty level: Easy **Preparation time:** 15 minutes

Cooking time: 28 minutes

Servings: 4

Ingredients:

- 1 cup finely shredded parsnips, steamed

- 8 oz ham, diced

- 2 eggs, beaten

- 1 ½ cups finely grated cheddar cheese

- ½ tsp garlic powder

- 2 tbsp chopped fresh parsley leaves

- ¼ tsp smoked paprika

- ½ tsp dried thyme

- Salt and freshly ground black pepper to taste

Directions:

1. Preheat the waffle iron.

2. In a medium bowl, mix all the ingredients.

3. Open the iron, lightly grease with cooking spray and pour in a quarter of the mixture.

4. Close the iron and cook until crispy, 7 minutes.

5. Remove the chaffle onto a plate and set aside.

6. Make three more chaffles using the remaining mixture.

7. Serve afterward.

Nutrition: Calories: 99 Cal Total Fat: 8 g Saturated Fat: 0 g Cholesterol: 0 mg Sodium: 0 mg Total Carbs: 4 g

6. <u>Cauliflower Turkey Chaffle</u>

Difficulty level: Medium

Preparation Time: 5 minutes

Cooking Time: 12 minutes

Servings: 2

Ingredients:

- One large egg (beaten)

- ½ cup cauliflower rice

- ¼ cup diced turkey

- ½ tsp coconut amino or soy sauce

- A pinch of ground black pepper

- A pinch of white pepper

- ¼ tsp curry

- ¼ tsp oregano

- 1 tbsp butter (melted)

- ¾ cup shredded mozzarella cheese

- One garlic clove (crushed)

Directions:

1. Plug the waffle maker to preheat it and spray it with a non-stick spray.

2. In a mixing bowl, combine the cauliflower rice, white pepper, black pepper, curry, and oregano.

3. In another mixing bowl, whisk together the eggs, butter, crushed garlic, and coconut amino. Pour the egg mixture into the cheese mixture and mix until the ingredients are well combined.

4. Add the diced turkey and stir to combine.

5. Sprinkle 2 tbsp cheese over the waffle maker. Fill the waffle maker with an appropriate amount of the batter. Spread out the mixture to the edges to cover all the holes on the waffle maker. Sprinkle another 2 tbsp cheese over the dough.

6. Close the waffle maker and cook for about 4 minutes or according to the waffle maker's settings.

7. After the cooking cycle, use a plastic or silicone utensil to remove the chaffle from the waffle maker.

8. Repeat steps 6 to 8 until you have cooked all the batter into chaffless.

9. Serve warm and enjoy.

Nutrition: Servings: 2 Amount per serving   Calories 168% Daily Value* Total Fat 11.5g 15% Saturated Fat 6.1g 30% Cholesterol 127mg 42% Sodium 184mg 8% Total Carbohydrate 3.8g 1% Dietary Fiber 0.2g 1% Total Sugars 1.2g Protein 12.5g   Vitamin D 13mcg 64% Calcium 30mg 2% Iron 2mg 13% Potassium 101mg 2%

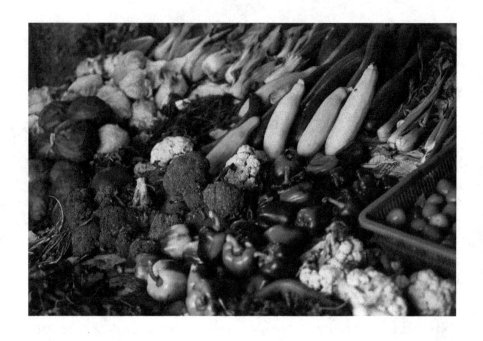

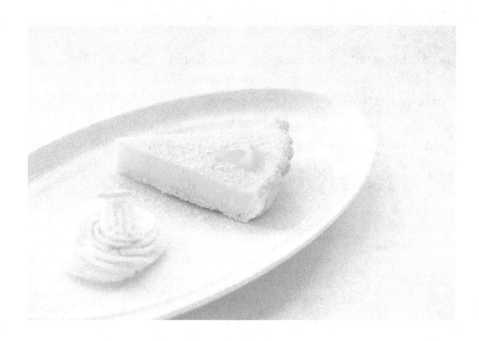

CHAPTER 2:

LUNCH CHAFFLE RECIPES

7. <u>Chicken And Chaffles</u>

Difficulty level: Medium

Preparation Time: 30 minutes   **Cooking Time:** 40 minutes **Servings:** 1 large chaffles or 2 mini chaffles

Ingredients

- Classic chaffle recipe or sweet chaffle recipe

- Keto fried chicken ingredients

- 2 boneless skinless chicken thighs

- Oil for frying

Egg wash ingredients

- 2 large eggs, whole

- 2 tbsp of heavy whipping cream

- Keto breading ingredients

- 2/3 cup of blanched almond flour

- 2/3 cup of grated parmesan cheese

- 1 tsp of salt

- 1/2 tsp of black pepper

- 1/2 tsp of paprika

  - 1/2 tsp of cayenne

Tools: waffle maker, mini or regular sized, three mixing bowls, measuring cups and tablespoons, spatula, non-stick cooking spray (or butter), pot for frying, blender, electric beaters, or whisk.

Directions

1. Pour 1-3 inches of oil into a pot on high heat.

2. Have the oil heat up to 350 degrees f.

3. While the oil is heating, take a bowl and mix the eggs and heavy cream until well mixed. Set aside.

4. Take another bowl and mix together the breading ingredients. Set aside.

5. Take each thawed chicken thigh and cut into 3-4 evenly sized pieces.

6. Dip each chicken slice in the breading, followed by dipping the slice in the egg wash, and then back in the breading again.

7. Make sure each side is evenly coated with breading.

8. Then dip the chicken slices slowly and carefully into the hot oil.

9. Keep the chicken slices in the oil until the slices are a deep brown and cooked through. About 5-7 minutes.

10. Do only a few slices at a time to avoid overcrowding the pot.

11. Follow the classic chaffle recipe.

12. Serve the chaffles and chicken on a plate and add some sugar-free pancake syrup or hot sauce to

13. taste.

14. Enjoy!

Nutrition: Calories 273, Carbs 6 g, Fat 11 g, Protein 37 g, Sodium 714 mg, Sugar 0 g

8. <u>Chaffle Cheese Sandwich</u>

Preparation time: 10 minutes

Difficulty level: Medium

Servings: 1

Cooking Time: 10 Minutes

Ingredients:

- 2 square keto chaffle

- 2 slice cheddar cheese

- 2 lettuce leaves

Directions:

1. Prepare your oven on 4000 F.

2. Arrange lettuce leave and cheese slice between chaffles.

3. Bake in the preheated oven for about 4-5 minutes Utes until cheese is melted.

4. Once the cheese is melted, remove from the oven.

5. Serve and enjoy!

Nutrition: Protein: 28% kcal Fat: 69% 149 kcal Carbohydrates: 3% 6 kcal

9. <u>Lox Bagel Chaffle</u>

Preparation Time: 30 minutes **Difficulty level:** Easy

Cooking Time: 40 minutes

Servings: 1 large chaffles or 2 mini chaffles

Ingredients

- Classic chaffle recipe or sweet chaffle recipe

- 2 tbsps of everything bagel seasoning

Filling ingredients

- 1 ounce of cream cheese

- 1 beefsteak tomato, thinly sliced

- 4-6 ounces of salmon gravlax

- 1 small shallot, thinly sliced

- Capers   1 tbsp of fresh dill

Tools: waffle maker, mini or regular sized, one mixing bowl, measuring cups and tablespoons, spatula, non-stick cooking spray (or butter), blender, electric beaters, or whisk.

Directions

1. Slice the tomato and the shallots.

2. Follow the classic chaffle recipe and everything bagel seasoning.

3. Once the chaffles are done, sprinkle more everything bagel seasoning onto the tops of both chaffles.

4. Lay two chaffles side by side and layer on the cream cheese, salmon, and shallots.

5. Sprinkle dill and capers and sandwich the two chaffles together.

6.   Enjoy!

Nutrition: Calories 203, Carbs 4.7 g, Fat 10 g, Protein 25 g, Sodium 479 mg, Sugar 0 g

CHAPTER 3:

DINNER CHAFFLES

10. Chicken Parmesan Chaffle

Difficulty level: Easy **Preparation Time:** 5 minutes

Cooking Time: 13 minutes **Servings:** 2

Ingredients:

- 1 egg (beaten)

- ½ cup shredded chicken

- 2 tbsp shredded parmesan cheese

- 1/3 cup shredded mozzarella cheese

- ¼ tsp garlic powder

- ¼ tsp onion powder 2 tbsp marinara sauce

- 1 tsp Italian seasoning

Garnish:

- 1 tbsp chopped green onions

Directions:

1. Plug the waffle maker to preheat it and spray it with a non-stick cooking spray. In a mixing bowl, combine the mozzarella cheese, shredded chicken, Italian seasoning, onion powder, and garlic powder. Add the egg and mix until the ingredients are well combined.

2. Pour half of the batter into the waffle maker and spread out the mixture to the edges to cover all the holes on the waffle maker. Close the waffle maker and cook for about 4 minutes or according to your waffle maker's settings. Meanwhile, preheat your oven to 400°F and line a baking sheet with parchment paper. After the cooking cycle, use a plastic or silicone utensil to remove the chaffle from the waffle maker.

3. Repeat 3, 4 and 6 to make the second chaffle.

4. Spread marinara sauce over the surface of both chaffless and sprinkle the parmesan cheese over the chaffless.

5. Arrange the chaffless into the baking sheet and place them in the oven—Bake for about 5 minutes or until the cheese melts. Remove the chaffless from the oven and let them cool for a few minutes. Serve and top with chopped green onion.

Nutrition: Servings: 2 Amount per serving Calories 144 % Daily Value* Total Fat 6.7g 9% Saturated Fat 2.7g 14% Cholesterol 118mg 39% Sodium 212mg 9% Total Carbohydrate 3.7g 1% Dietary Fiber 0.5g 2% Total Sugars 2g Protein 16.9g Vitamin D 8mcg 39% Calcium 89mg 7% Iron 1mg 5% Potassium 160mg 3%

CHAPTER 4:

CHAFFLE CAKE &

SANDWICH RECIPES

11. Chocolate Chaffle Cake

Preparation time: 6 minutes

Difficulty level: EASY **Servings:** 2

Cooking Time: 8 Minutes

Ingredients:

- Chocolate Chaffle Cake Ingredients:

- 2 tablespoons cocoa powder

- 2 tablespoons Swerve granulated sweetener

- 1 egg

- 1 tablespoon heavy whipping cream

- 1 tablespoon almond flour

- 1/4 tsp baking powder

- 1/2 tsp vanilla extract

- Cream Cheese Frosting:

- 2 tablespoons cream cheese

- 2 teaspoons swerve confectioners

- 1/8 tsp vanilla extract

- 1 tsp heavy cream

Directions:

1. How to Make Chocolate Chaffle Cake: In a small bowl, whisk together cocoa powder, swerve, almond flour, and baking powder. Add in the vanilla extract and heavy whipping cream and mix well.

2. Add in the egg and mix well. Be sure to scrape the sides of the bowl to get all of the ingredients mixed well.

3. Let sit for 3-4 minutes while the mini waffle maker heats up.

4. Add half of the waffle mixture to the waffle maker and cook for 4 minutes. Then cook the second waffle. While the second chocolate keto waffle is cooking, make your frosting. How to Make Cream Cheese Frosting:

5. In a small microwave-safe bowl add 2 tablespoons cream cheese. Microwave the cream cheese for seconds to soften the cream cheese.

6. Add in heavy whipping cream and vanilla extract and use a small hand mixer to mix well.

7. Then add in the confectioners swerve and use the hand mixer to incorporate and fluffy the frosting.

8. Assembling Keto Chocolate Chaffle cake: Place one chocolate chaffle on a plate, top with a layer of frosting. You can spread it with a knife or use a pastry bag and pipe the frosting.

9. Put the second chocolate chaffle on top of the frosting layer and then spread or pipe the rest of the frosting on top.

Nutrition: (per serving):Calories: 151kcal ;Carbohydrates:5g ;Protein: 6g;Fat: 13g ;Saturated Fat:6g ;Cholesterol:111mg ;Sodium:83mg ;Potassium: 190mg ;Fiber: 2g ;Sugar: 1g ;Vitamin A: 461IU ;Calcium: 67mg ;Iron: 1mg

12. Tomato Sandwich Chaffles

Preparation time: 6 minutes

Difficulty level: EASY

Servings: 2

Cooking Time: 6 Minutes

Ingredients:

- Chaffles

- 1 large organic egg, beaten

- ½ cup colby jack cheese, shredded finely

- 1/8 teaspoon organic vanilla extract

- Filling

- 1 small tomato, sliced

- 2 teaspoons fresh basil leaves

Directions:

1. Preheat a mini waffle iron and then grease it.

2. For chaffles: in a small bowl, place all the ingredients and stir to combine.

3. Place half of the mixture into preheated waffle iron and cook for about minutes.

4. Repeat with the remaining mixture.

5. Serve each chaffle with tomato slices and basil leaves.

Nutrition: Calories 155 Net Carbs 2.4 g Total Fat 11.g Saturated Fat 6.8 g Cholesterol 118 mg Sodium 217 mg Total Carbs 3 g Fiber 0.6 g Sugar 1.4 g Protein 9.6 g

13.Chocolate Sandwich Chaffles

Preparation time: 6 minutes

Difficulty level: EASY

Servings: 2

Cooking Time: 10 Minutes

Ingredients:

- Chaffles

- 1 organic egg, beaten

- 1 ounce cream cheese, softened

- 2 tablespoons almond flour

- 1 tablespoon cacao powder

- 2 teaspoons erythritol

- 1 teaspoon organic vanilla extract

- Filling 2 tablespoons cream cheese, softened

- 2 tablespoons erythritol

- ½ tablespoon cacao powder

- ¼ teaspoon organic vanilla extract

Directions:

1. Preheat a mini waffle iron and then grease it. For chaffles: In a medium bowl, put all ingredients and with a fork, mix until well combined. Place half of the mixture into preheated waffle iron and cook for about 3–5 minutes. Repeat with the remaining mixture.

2. Meanwhile, for filling: In a medium bowl, put all ingredients and with a hand mixer, beat until well combined.

3. Serve each chaffle with chocolate mixture.

Nutrition: Calories 192 Net Carb: g Total Fat 16 g Saturated Fat 7.6 g Cholesterol 113 mg Sodium 115 mg Total Carbs 4.4 g Fiber 1.9 g Sugar 0.8 g Protein 5.7 g

CHAPTER 5:

VEGETARIAN CHAFFLE

RECIPES

14.Cheesy Garlic Chaffle Bread Recipe

Preparation time: 10 minutes

Difficulty level: Hard

Cooking Time: 14 Minutes

Servings: 2

Ingredients:

- 1 egg

- 1/2 cup mozzarella cheese, shredded

- 1 tbsp parmesan cheese

- 3/4 tsp coconut flour

- 1/4 tsp baking powder

- 1/8 tsp Italian Seasoning

- Pinch of salt

- 1 tbsp butter, melted

- 1/4 tsp garlic powder

- 1/2 cup mozzarella cheese, shredded

- 1/4 tsp basil seasoning

Directions:

1. Preheat oven to 400 degrees. Plug the Dash Mini Waffle Maker in the wall and allow it to get hot. Lightly grease waffle maker.

2. Combine the first 7 ingredients in a small bowl and stir well to combine.

3. Spoon half of the batter on the waffle maker and close — Cook for 4 minutes or until golden brown.

4. Remove the chaffle bread carefully from the Dash Mini Waffle Maker, then repeat for the rest of the batter.

5. In a small bowl, melt the butter and add garlic powder.

6. Cut each chaffle in half (or thirds), and place on a baking sheet, then brush the tops with the garlic butter mixture.

7. Top with mozzarella cheese and pop in the oven for 4 -5 minutes.

8. Turn oven to broil and move the baking pan to the top shelf for 1-2 minutes so that the cheese begins to bubble and turn golden brown. Watch

very carefully, as it can burn quickly on broil. (check every 30 seconds)

9. Remove from oven and sprinkle basil seasoning on top. Enjoy!

Nutrition: (per serving):Calories: 270kcal ;Carbohydrates:3g ;Protein: 16g;Fat: 21g ;Saturated Fat:12g;Fiber: 1g ;Sugar: 1g

CHAPTER 6:

BASIC CHAFFLES RECIPES

15. Cranberry And Brie Chaffle

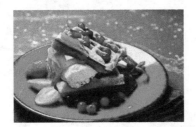

Preparation time: 10 minutes **Difficulty level:** Medium

Cooking time: 20 minutes **Servings:** 4 mini chaffles

Ingredients:

- 4 tablespoons frozen cranberries

- 3 tablespoons swerve sweetener

- 1 cup / 115 grams shredded brie cheese

- 2 eggs, at room temperature

Directions:

1. Take a non-stick waffle iron, plug it in, select the medium or medium-high heat setting and let it preheat until ready to use; it could also be indicated with an indicator light changing its color.

2. Meanwhile, prepare the batter and for this, take a heatproof bowl, add cheese in it, and microwave at high heat setting for 15 seconds or until cheese has softened. Then add sweetener, berries, and egg into the cheese and whisk with an electric mixer until smooth. Use a ladle to pour one-fourth of the prepared batter into the heated waffle iron in a spiral direction, starting from the edges, then shut the lid and cook for 4 minutes or more until solid and nicely browned; the cooked waffle will look like a cake.

3. When done, transfer chaffles to a plate with a silicone spatula and repeat with the remaining batter.

4. Let chaffles stand for some time until crispy and serve straight away.

Nutrition: Calories 320 Carbohydrates 2.9 g Protein 21.5 g Fat 24.3g

16.Bacon & Cheddar Cheese Chaffles

Preparation time: 5 minutes

Difficulty level: Medium

Cooking time: 5 minutes

Servings: 6

Ingredients:

- ½ cup almond flour

- 3 bacon strips

- ¼ cup sour cream

- 1 ½ cup cheddar cheese

- ½ cup smoked Gouda cheese

- ½ tsp onion powder

- ½ tsp. baking powder

- ¼ cup oat

- 1 egg

- 1 tbsp. oil

- 1 ½ tbsp. butter

- ¼ tsp. salt

- ½ tsp. parsley

- ¼ tsp. baking soda

Directions:

1. Heat the waffle maker. Take a bowl add almond flour, baking powder, baking soda, onion powder, garlic salt and mix well. In another bowl whisk eggs, bacon, cream, parsley, butter and cheese until well combined.

2. Now pour the mixture over dry ingredients and mix well.

3. Pour the batter over the preheated waffle maker and cook for 5 to 6 minutes or until golden brown. Serve the hot and crispy chaffles.

Nutrition: Calories 320 Carbohydrates 2.9 g Protein 21.5 g Fat 24.3g

17.White Bread Keto Chaffle

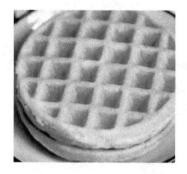

Preparation time: 5 minutes

Difficulty level: Medium

Cooking time: 4 minutes

Servings: 2

Ingredients

- 2 egg whites

- Cream cheese, melted

- 2 tsp water

- 1/4 tsp baking powder

- 1/4 cup almond flour

- 1 Pinch of salt

Directions

1. Pre-heat the mini waffle maker,

2. Whisk the egg whites together with the cream cheese and water in a bowl.

3. Next step is to add the baking powder, almond flour and salt and whisk until you have a smooth batter. Then you pour half of the batter into the mini waffle maker.

4. Allow to cook for roughly 4 minutes or until you no longer see steam coming from the waffle maker.

5. Remove and allow to cool.

Nutrition: Calories 320 Carbohydrates 2.9 g Protein 21.5 g Fat 24.3g

18.Banana Foster Chaffle

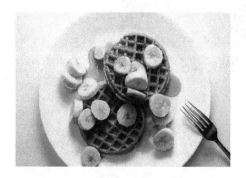

Preparation time: 10 minutes

Difficulty level: Medium **Cooking time:** 20 minutes

Servings: 4 large chaffles

Ingredients:

For Chaffle:

- 1/8 teaspoon cinnamon

- ½ teaspoon banana extract, unsweetened

- 4 teaspoons swerve sweetener

- 1 cup / 225 grams cream cheese, softened

- ½ teaspoon vanilla extract, unsweetened

- 8 eggs, at room temperature

For Syrup:

- 20 drops of banana extract, unsweetened

- 8 teaspoons swerve sweetener

- 20 drops of caramel extract, unsweetened

- 12 drops of rum extract, unsweetened

- 8 tablespoons unsalted butter

- 1/8 teaspoon cinnamon

Directions:

1. Take a non-stick waffle iron, plug it in, select the medium or medium-high heat setting and let it preheat until ready to use; it could also be indicated with an indicator light changing its color.

2. Meanwhile, prepare the batter for chaffle and for this, take a large bowl, crack eggs in it, add sweetener, cream cheese, and all the extracts and then mix with an electric mixer until smooth, let the batter stand for 5 minutes.

3. Use a ladle to pour one-fourth of the prepared batter into the heated waffle iron in a spiral direction, starting from the edges, then shut the lid and cook for 5 minutes or more until solid and nicely browned; the cooked waffle will look like a cake.

4. When done, transfer chaffles to a plate with a silicone spatula, repeat with the remaining batter and let chaffles stand for some time until crispy.

5. Meanwhile, prepare the syrup and for this, take a small heatproof bowl, add butter in it, and microwave at high heat setting for 15 seconds until it melts.

6. Then add remaining ingredients for the syrup and mix until combined.

7. Drizzle syrup over chaffles and then serve.

Nutrition: Calories 320 Carbohydrates 2.9 g Fat 24.3g

CHAPTER 7:

SWEET CHAFFLES RECIPES

19.Chocolate Chip Chaffles

Preparation time: 8 minutes

Difficulty level: Medium

Servings: 1

Cooking Time: 6 Minutes

Ingredients:

- 1 egg

- 1 tsp coconut flour

- 1 tsp sweetener

- ½ tsp vanilla extract

- ¼ cup heavy whipping cream, for serving

- ½ cup almond milk ricotta, finely shredded

- 2 tbsp sugar-free chocolate chips

Directions:

1. Preheat your mini waffle iron.

2. Mix the egg, coconut flour, vanilla, and sweetener. Whisk together with a fork. Stir in the almond milk ricotta.

3. Pour half of the batter into the waffle iron and dot with a pinch of chocolate chips.

4. Close the waffle iron and cook for minutes. Repeat with remaining batter.

5. Serve hot with the whipped cream.

Nutrition: Calories per Servings: 304 Kcal, Fats: 16 g ,Carbs: 7 g ,Protein: 3 g

20. <u>Red Velvet Chaffles</u>

Preparation time: 5 minutes

Difficulty level: Medium

Cooking Time: 8 Minutes

Servings: 2

Ingredients:

- 2 tablespoons cacao powder

- 2 tablespoons erythritol

- 1 organic egg, beaten

- 2 drops super red food coloring

- ¼ teaspoon organic baking powder

- 1 tablespoon heavy whipping cream

Directions:

1. Preheat a mini waffle iron and then grease it.

2. In a medium bowl, put all ingredients and with a fork, mix until well combined. Place half of the

mixture into preheated waffle iron and cook for about 4 minutes.

3. Repeat with the remaining mixture.

4. Serve warm.

Nutrition: Calories 70 Net Carbs 1.7 g Total Fat g Saturated Fat 3 g Cholesterol 92 mg Sodium 34 mg Total Carbs 3.2 g Fiber 1.5 g Sugar 0.2 g Protein 3.9 g

21.Almond Butter Chaffles

Preparation time: 5 minutes

Difficulty level: Medium

Cooking Time: 10 Minutes

Servings: 2

Ingredients:

- 1 large organic egg, beaten

- 1/3 cup Mozzarella cheese, shredded

- 1 tablespoon Erythritol

- 2 tablespoons almond butter

- 1 teaspoon organic vanilla extract

Directions:

1. Preheat a mini waffle iron and then grease it.

2. In a medium bowl, place all ingredients and with a fork, mix until well combined.

3. Place half of the mixture into preheated waffle iron and cook for about 5 minutes or until golden brown. Repeat with the remaining mixture.

4. Serve warm.

Nutrition: Calories: 153Net Carb: 2gFat: 12.3gSaturated Fat: 2gCarbohydrates: 3.Dietary Fiber: 1.6g Sugar: 1.2gProtein: 7.9g

22. <u>Chocolate Chips Chaffles</u>

Preparation time: 5 minutes

Difficulty level: Medium

Cooking Time: 8 Minutes **Servings:** 2

Ingredients:

- 1 large organic egg

- 1 teaspoon coconut flour

- 1 teaspoon Erythritol

- ½ teaspoon organic vanilla extract

- ½ cup Mozzarella cheese, shredded finely

- 2 tablespoons 70% dark chocolate chips

Directions:

1. Preheat a mini waffle iron and then grease it. In a bowl, place the egg, coconut flour, sweetener and vanilla extract and beat until well combined.

2. Add the cheese and stir to combine.

3. Place half of the mixture into preheated waffle iron and top with half of the chocolate chips.

4. Place a little egg mixture over each chocolate chip. Cook for about 3-4 minutes or until golden brown.

5. Repeat with the remaining mixture and chocolate chips.

6. Serve warm.

Nutrition: Calories: 164Net Carb: 2.Fat: 11.9gSaturated Fat: 6.6gCarbohydrates: 5.4gDietary Fiber: 2.5g Sugar: 0.3gProtein: 7.3g

23. <u>Peanut Butter Chaffles</u>

Preparation time: 5 minutes

Difficulty level: Medium **Time:** 8 Minutes

Cooking Time: 10 minutes

Servings: 2

Ingredients:

- 1 organic egg, beaten

- ½ cup Mozzarella cheese, shredded

- 3 tablespoons granulated Erythritol

- 2 tablespoons peanut butter

Directions:

1. Preheat a mini waffle iron and then grease it.

2. In a medium bowl, place all ingredients and with a fork, mix until well combined.

3. Place half of the mixture into preheated waffle iron and cook for about 4 minutes or until golden brown.

4. Repeat with the remaining mixture.

5. Serve warm.

Nutrition: Calories: 145Net Carb: 2.Fat: 11.5gSaturated Fat: 3.1gCarbohydrates: 3.6gDietary Fiber: 1g Sugar: 1.7gProtein: 8.8g

CHAPTER 8:

DESSERT CHAFFLES

24. <u>Raspberry And Chocolate Chaffle</u>

Preparation time: 5 minutes

Difficulty level: Hard

Cooking Time: 7–9 Minutes

Servings: 2

Ingredients:

- Batter

- 4 eggs

- 2 ounces cream cheese, softened

- 2 ounces sour cream

- 1 teaspoon vanilla extract

- 5 tablespoons almond flour

- ¼ cup cocoa powder

- 1½ teaspoons baking powder

- 2 ounces fresh or frozen raspberries

- Other

- 2 tablespoons butter to brush the waffle maker

- Fresh sprigs of mint to garnish

Directions:

1. Preheat the waffle maker.

2. Add the eggs, cream cheese and sour cream to a bowl and stir with a wire whisk until just combined.

3. Add the vanilla extract and mix until combined.

4. Stir in the almond flour, cocoa powder, and baking powder and mix until combined.

5. Add the raspberries and stir until combined.

6. Brush the heated waffle maker with butter and add a few tablespoons of the batter.

7. Close the lid and cook for about 8 minutes depending on your waffle maker.

8. Serve with fresh sprigs of mint.

Nutrition: Calories 270, fat 23 g, carbs 8.g, sugar 1.3 g, Protein 10.2 g, sodium 158 mg

25. <u>Chicken Chaffle Sandwich</u>

Preparation time: 10 minutes

Difficulty level: Hard

Cooking Time: 15 Minutes

Servings: 2

Ingredients:

- 1 chicken breast fillet, sliced into strips

- Salt and pepper to taste

- 1 teaspoon dried rosemary

- 1 tablespoon olive oil

- 4 basic chaffles

- 2 tablespoons butter, melted

- 2 tablespoons Parmesan cheese, grated

Directions:

1. Season the chicken strips with salt, pepper and rosemary.

2. Add olive oil to a pan over medium low heat.

3. Cook the chicken until brown on both sides.

4. Spread butter on top of each chaffle.

5. Sprinkle cheese on top.

6. Place the chicken on top and top with another chaffle.

Nutrition: Calories 262 Total Fat 20g Saturated Fat 9.2g Cholesterol mg Sodium 270mg Potassium 125mg Total Carbohydrate 1g Dietary Fiber 0.2g Protein 20.2g Total Sugars 0g

26. <u>Christmas Smoothie With Chaffles</u>

Preparation time: 10 minutes

Difficulty level: Hard

Cooking Time:0 Minutes

Servings: 2

Ingredients:

- 1 cup coconut milk

- 2 tbsps. almonds chopped

- ¼ cup cherries

- 1 pinch sea salt

- 1/4 cup ice cubes

- FOR TOPPING

- 2 oz. keto chocolate chips

- 2 oz. cherries

- 2 minutes chaffles

- 2 scoop heavy cream, frozen

Directions:

1. Add almond milk, almonds, cherries, salt and ice in a blender, blend for 2 minutes Utes until smooth and fluffy. Pour the smoothie into glasses.

2. Top with one scoop heavy cream, chocolate chips, cherries and chaffle in each glass. Serve and enjoy!

Nutrition: Protein: 4% 11 kcal Fat: 84% 24kcal Carbohydrates: 13% 37 kcal

27. Quick & Easy Blueberry Chaffle

Preparation time: 10 minutes

Difficulty level: Hard

Cooking Time: 15 Minutes

Servings: 2

Ingredients:

- 1 egg, lightly beaten

- 1/4 cup blueberries

- 1/2 tsp vanilla

- 1 oz cream cheese

- 1/4 tsp baking powder, gluten-free

- 4 tsp Swerve

- 1 tbsp coconut flour

Directions:

1. Preheat your waffle maker.

2. In a small bowl, mix coconut flour, baking powder, and Swerve until well combined.

3. Add vanilla, cream cheese, egg, and vanilla and whisk until combined.

4. Spray waffle maker with cooking spray.

5. Pour half batter in the hot waffle maker and top with 4-blueberries and cook for 4-5 minutes until golden brown. Repeat with the remaining batter. Serve and enjoy.

Nutrition: Calories 135Fat 8.2 carbohydrates 11 sugar 2.6 protein 5 cholesterol 9mg

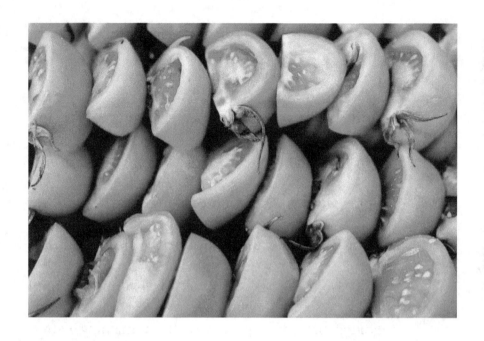

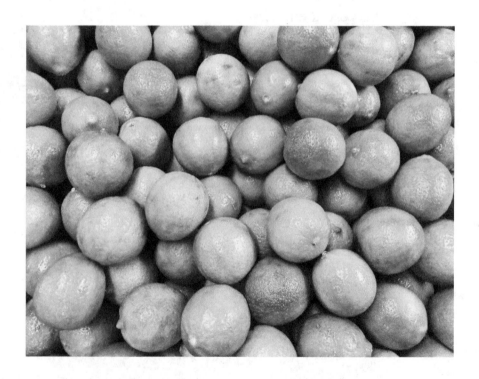

CHAPTER 9:

SAVORY CHAFFLES

RECIPES

28. Jalapeño Chaffles

Preparation time: 6 minutes

Difficulty level: Easy

Cooking Time: 10 Minutes **Servings:** 2

Ingredients:

- 1 organic egg, beaten

- ½ cup Cheddar cheese, shredded

- ½ tablespoon jalapeño pepper, chopped

- Salt, to taste

Directions:

1. Preheat a mini waffle iron and then grease it. In a medium bowl, place all ingredients and with a fork, mix until well combined.

2. Place half of the mixture into preheated waffle iron and cook for about 5 minutes or until golden brown.

3. Repeat with the remaining mixture.

4. Serve warm.

Nutrition: Calories: 14et Carb: 0.6gFat: 11.6gSaturated Fat: 6.6gCarbohydrates: 0.6gDietary Fiber: 0g Sugar: 0.4gProtein: 9.8g

29. Bbq Rub Chaffles

Preparation time: 10 minutes

Difficulty level: Easy

Cooking Time: 20 Minutes

Servings: 2

Ingredients:

- 2 organic eggs, beaten

- 1 cup Cheddar cheese, shredded

- ½ teaspoon BBQ rub

- ¼ teaspoon organic baking powder

Directions:

1. Preheat a mini waffle iron and then grease it. In a medium bowl, place all ingredients and with a fork, mix until well combined. Place ¼ of the mixture into preheated waffle iron and cook for about 5 minutes or until golden brown.

2. Repeat with the remaining mixture.

3. Serve warm.

Nutrition: Calories: 14et Carb: 0.7gFat: 11.6gSaturated Fat: 6.6gCarbohydrates: 0.7gDietary Fiber: 0g Sugar: 0.3gProtein: 9.8g

30. Bagel Seasoning Chaffles

Preparation time: 10 minutes

Difficulty level: Easy

Cooking Time: 20 Minutes **Servings:** 2

Ingredients:

- 1 large organic egg

- 1 cup Mozzarella cheese, shredded

- 1 tablespoon almond flour

- 1 teaspoon organic baking powder

- 2 teaspoons bagel seasoning

- ¼ teaspoon garlic powder

- ¼ teaspoon onion powder

Directions:

1. Preheat a mini waffle iron and then grease it.

2. In a medium bowl, place all ingredients and with a fork, mix until well combined.

3. Place ¼ of the mixture into preheated waffle iron and cook for about 4 minutes or until golden brown.

4. Repeat with the remaining mixture.

5. Serve warm.

Nutrition: Calories: 73Net Carb: 2gFat: 5.5gSaturated Fat: 1.5gCarbohydrates: 2.3gDietary Fiber: 0.3g Sugar: 0.9gProtein: 3.7g

31.Avocado Chaffle

Preparation time: 6 minutes

Cooking Time: 10 Minutes

Difficulty level: Easy

Servings: 2

Ingredients:

- ½ avocado, sliced

- ½ tsp lemon juice

- ⅛ tsp salt

- ⅛ tsp black pepper

- 1 egg ½ cup shredded cheese

- ¼ crumbled feta cheese

- 1 cherry tomato, halved

Directions:

1. Mash together avocado, lemon juice, salt, and pepper until well-combined.

2. Turn on waffle maker to heat and oil it with cooking spray.

3. Beat egg in a small mixing bowl.

4. Place ⅛ cup of cheese on waffle maker, then spread half of the egg mixture over it and top with ⅛ cup of cheese.

5. Close and cook for 3-4 minutes. Repeat for remaining batter.

6. Let chaffles cool for 3-4 minutes, then spread avocado mix on top of each.

7. Top with crumbled feta and cherry tomato halves.

Nutrition: Carbs: 5 g ;Fat: 19 g ;Protein: 7 g ;Calories: 232

32. <u>Cheddar Jalapeño Chaffle</u>

Preparation time: 6 minutes

Difficulty level: Hard

Cooking Time: 5 Minutes

Servings: 2

Ingredients:

- 2 large eggs

- ½ cup shredded mozzarella

- ¼ cup almond flour

- ½ tsp baking powder

- ¼ cup shredded cheddar cheese

- 2 Tbsp diced jalapeños jarred or canned

- For the toppings:

- ½ cooked bacon, chopped

- 2 Tbsp cream cheese

- ¼ jalapeño slices

Directions:

1. Turn on waffle maker to heat and oil it with cooking spray.

2. Mix mozzarella, eggs, baking powder, almond flour, and garlic powder in a bowl.

3. Sprinkle 2 Tbsp cheddar cheese in a thin layer on waffle maker, and ½ jalapeño.

4. Ladle half of the egg mixture on top of the cheese and jalapeños.

5. Cook for minutes, or until done.

6. Repeat for the second chaffle.

7. Top with cream cheese, bacon, and jalapeño slices.

Nutrition: Carbs: 5 g ;Fat: 1g ;Protein: 18 g ;Calories: 307

33. **3-Cheeses Herbed Chaffles**

Preparation time: 10 minutes

Difficulty level: Easy

Cooking Time: 12 Minutes **Servings:** 2

Ingredients:

- 4 tablespoons almond flour

- 1 tablespoon coconut flour

- 1 teaspoon mixed dried herbs

- ½ teaspoon organic baking powder

- ¼ teaspoon garlic powder

- ¼ teaspoon onion powder

- Salt and freshly ground black pepper, to taste

- ¼ cup cream cheese, softened

- 3 large organic eggs

- ½ cup Cheddar cheese, grated

- 1/3 cup Parmesan cheese, grated

Directions:

1. Preheat a waffle iron and then grease it.

2. In a bowl, mix together the flours, dried herbs, baking powder and seasoning and mix well.

3. In a separate bowl, put cream cheese and eggs and beat until well combined.

4. Add the flour mixture, cheddar and Parmesan cheese and mix until well combined.

5. Place the desired amount of the mixture into preheated waffle iron and cook for about 2-3 minutes or until golden brown.

6. Repeat with the remaining mixture.

7. Serve warm.

Nutrition: Calories: 240Net Carb: 2.6gFat: 19gSaturated Fat: 5gCarbohydrates: 4gDietary Fiber: 1.6g Sugar: 0.7gProtein: 12.3g

34. <u>Zucchini Chaffles</u>

Preparation time: 10 minutes

Difficulty level: Easy

Cooking Time: 18 Minutes

Servings: 2

Ingredients:

- 2 large zucchinis, grated and squeezed

- 2 large organic eggs

- 2/3 cup Cheddar cheese, shredded

- 2 tablespoons coconut flour

- ½ teaspoon garlic powder

- ½ teaspoon red pepper flakes, crushed

- Salt, to taste

Directions:

1. Preheat a waffle iron and then grease it.

2. In a medium bowl, place all ingredients and, mix until well combined.

3. Place ¼ of the mixture into preheated waffle iron and cook for about 4-4½ minutes or until golden brown.

4. Repeat with the remaining mixture.

5. Serve warm.

Nutrition: Calories: 159Net Carb: 4.3gFat: 10gSaturated Fat: 5.8gCarbohydrates: 8gDietary Fiber: 3.7g Sugar: 2.Protein: 10.1g

CHAPTER 10:

FESTIVE CHAFFLE

RECIPES

35. <u>Chaffles And Ice-Cream Platter</u>

Preparation time: 10 minutes

Cooking Time: 5 minutes

Difficulty level: Medium

Servings: 2

Ingredients:

- 2 keto brownie chaffles

- 2 scoop vanilla keto ice cream

- 8 oz. strawberries, sliced

- keto chocolate sauce

Directions:

1. Arrange chaffles, ice-cream, strawberries slice in serving plate.

2. Drizzle chocolate sauce on top.

3. Serve and enjoy!

Nutrition: Protein: 26% kcal Fat: 68% 128 kcal Carbohydrates: 6% 11 kcal

36. <u>Thanksgiving Pumpkin Spice Chaffle</u>

Preparation time: 5 minutes

Difficulty level: Medium

Cooking Time: 5minutes

Servings: 2

Ingredients:

- 1 cup egg whites

- ¼ cup pumpkin puree

- 2 tsps. pumpkin pie spice

- 2 tsps. coconut flour

- ½ tsp. vanilla

- 1 tsp. baking powder

- 1 tsp. baking soda

- 1/8 tsp cinnamon powder

- 1 cup mozzarella cheese, grated

- 1/2 tsp. garlic powder

Directions:

1. Switch on your square waffle maker. Spray with non-stick spray.

2. Beat egg whites with beater, until fluffy and white.

3. Add pumpkin puree, pumpkin pie spice, coconut flour in egg whites and beat again.

4. Stir in the cheese, cinnamon powder, garlic powder, baking soda, and powder.

5. Pour ½ of the batter in the waffle maker.

6. Close the maker and cook for about 3 minutes Utes.

7. Repeat with the remaining batter.

8. Remove chaffles from the maker.

9. Serve hot and enjoy!

Nutrition: Protein: 51% 66 kcal Fat: 41% 53 kcal Carbohydrates: 8% kcal

37. <u>Cookie Dough Chaffle</u>

Preparation time: 5 minutes

Difficulty level: Medium

Cooking Time:7–9 Minutes

Servings: 2

Ingredients:

- Batter

- 4 eggs

- ¼ cup heavy cream

- 1 teaspoon vanilla extract

- ¼ cup stevia

- 6 tablespoons coconut flour

- 1 teaspoon baking powder

- Pinch of salt

- ¼ cup unsweetened chocolate chips

- Other

- 2 tablespoons cooking spray to brush the waffle maker

- ¼ cup heavy cream, whipped

Directions:

1. Preheat the waffle maker.

2. Add the eggs and heavy cream to a bowl and stir in the vanilla extract, stevia, coconut flour, baking powder, and salt. Mix until just combined.

3. Stir in the chocolate chips and combine.

4. Brush the heated waffle maker with cooking spray and add a few tablespoons of the batter.

5. Close the lid and cook for about 7–8 minutes depending on your waffle maker.

6. Serve with whipped cream on top.

Nutrition: Calories 3, fat 32.3 g, carbs 12.6 g, sugar 0.5 g, Protein 9 g, sodium 117 mg

38. Cinnamon And Vanilla Chaffle

Preparation time: 5 minutes

Difficulty level: Medium

Cooking Time:7–9 Minutes

Servings: 2

Ingredients:

- Batter

- 4 eggs

- 4 ounces sour cream

- 1 teaspoon vanilla extract

- 1 teaspoon cinnamon

- ¼ cup stevia

- 5 tablespoons coconut flour

- Other

- 2 tablespoons coconut oil to brush the waffle maker

- ½ teaspoon cinnamon for garnishing the chaffles

Directions:

1. Preheat the waffle maker.

2. Add the eggs and sour cream to a bowl and stir with a wire whisk until just combined.

3. Add the vanilla extract, cinnamon, and stevia and mix until combined.

4. Stir in the coconut flour and stir until combined.

5. Brush the heated waffle maker with coconut oil and add a few tablespoons of the batter.

6. Close the lid and cook for about 7–8 minutes depending on your waffle maker.

7. Serve and enjoy.

Nutrition: Calories 224, fat 11 g, carbs 8.4 g, sugar 0.5 g, Protein 7.7 g, sodium 77 mg

CHAPTER 11:

SPECIAL CHAFFLE

RECIPES

39. <u>New Year Keto Chaffle Cake</u>

Preparation Time: 5 Minutes

Servings: 5

Difficulty level: Medium

Cooking Time: 15 minutes

Ingredients:

- 4 oz. almond flour

- 2 cup cheddar cheese

- 5 eggs

- 1 tsp. stevia

- 2 tsp baking powder

- 2 tsp vanilla extract

- 1/4 cup almond butter, melted

- 3 tbsps. almond milk

- 1 cup cranberries

- I cup coconut cream

Directions:

1. Crack eggs in a small mixing bowl, mix the eggs, almond flour, stevia, and baking powder.

2. Add the melted butter slowly to the flour mixture, mix well to ensure a smooth consistency.

3. Add the cheese, almond milk, cranberries and vanilla to the flour and butter mixture be sure to mix well.

4. Preheat waffles maker according to manufacturer instruction and grease it with avocado oil.

5. Pour mixture into waffle maker and cook until golden brown.

6. Make 5 chaffles

7. Stag chaffles in a plate. Spread the cream all around.

8. Cut in slice and serve.

Nutrition: Protein: 3% 15 Kcal Fat: % 207 Kcal Carbohydrates: 3% 15 Kcal

40. <u>Swiss Bacon Chaffle</u>

Preparation time: 10 minutes   **Difficulty level:** Medium

Cooking Time: 8 Minutes **Servings:** 2

Ingredients:

- 1 egg

- ½ cup Swiss cheese

- 2 tablespoons cooked crumbled bacon

Directions:

1. Preheat your waffle maker. Beat the egg in a bowl.

2. Stir in the cheese and bacon.

3. Pour half of the mixture into the device.

4. Close and cook for 4 minutes.

5. Cook the second chaffle using the same steps.

Nutrition: Calories 23 Total Fat 17.6g Saturated Fat 8.1g Cholesterol128mg Sodium 522mg Total Carbohydrate 1.9g ietaryFiber 0g Total Sugars 0.5g Protein 17.1g Potassium 158mg

41.Pumpkin Chaffle With Frosting

Preparation time: 10 minutes

Difficulty level: Medium

Cooking Time: 15 Minutes

Servings: 2

Ingredients:

- 1 egg, lightly beaten

- 1 tbsp sugar-free pumpkin puree

- 1/4 tsp pumpkin pie spice

- 1/2 cup mozzarella cheese, shredded

- For frosting:

- 1/2 tsp vanilla

- 2 tbsp Swerve

- 2 tbsp cream cheese, softened

Directions:

1. Preheat your waffle maker.

2. Add egg in a bowl and whisk well.

3. Add pumpkin puree, pumpkin pie spice, and cheese and stir well.

4. Spray waffle maker with cooking spray.

5. Pour 1/2 of the batter in the hot waffle maker and cook for 3-4 minutes or until golden brown. Repeat with the remaining batter.

6. In a small bowl, mix all frosting ingredients until smooth.

7. Add frosting on top of hot chaffles and serve.

Nutrition: Calories 9at 7 carbohydrates 3.6 sugar 0.6 protein 5.6 cholesterol 97 mg

CHAPTER 12:

OTHER KETO CHAFFLES

42. Simple Heart Shape Chaffles

Preparation time: 25 minutes

Difficulty level: Easy

servings: 4

Cooking Time: 5 Minutes

Servings: 2

Ingredients:

- 2 large eggs

- 1 cup finely shredded mozzarella

- 2 tbsps. coconut flour

- 1 tsp. stevia

- Coconut flour for topping

Directions:

1. Switch on your heart shape Belgian waffle maker.

2. Grease with cooking spray and let it preheat.

3. Mix together chaffle ingredients in a mixing bowl.

4. Pour chaffle mixture in heart shape Belgian maker and cook for about 5 minutes Utes.

5. Once chaffles are cooked, carefully remove from the maker.

6. Sprinkle coconut flour on top.

7. Serve with warm keto BLT coffee.

8. Enjoy!

Nutrition: Protein: 32% 52 kcal Fat: 57% kcal Carbohydrates: 10% 17 kcal

43. <u>Chicken Jalapeno Popper Chaffle</u>

Preparation time: 9 minutes

Difficulty level: Easy

Cooking Time: 10 Minutes

Servings: 2

Ingredients:

- 1 egg

- 1 small jalapeno pepper (sliced)

- 1 can chicken breast (diced)

- A pinch of salt

- A pinch of ground black pepper

- 1/8 tsp garlic powder

- 1/8 tsp onion powder

- 2 tbsp shredded parmesan cheese

- 4 tbsp shredded cheddar cheese

- 1 tsp cream cheese

- Topping:

- Sour cream

Directions:

1. Plug the waffle maker to preheat it and spray it with a non-stick spray.

2. In a mixing bowl, combine parmesan, cheddar, jalapeno, salt, ground pepper, garlic powder and onion powder.

3. Whisk together the egg and cream cheese. Pour it into the cheese mixture and mix until the ingredients are well combined. Fold in the diced chicken.

4. Fill the waffle maker with about ½ of the batter and spread out the batter to cover all the holes on the waffle maker.

5. Close the waffle maker and cook for about minutes or according to waffle maker's settings.

6. After the cooking cycle, use a plastic or silicone utensil to remove the chaffle from the waffle maker.

7. Repeat step 4 to 6 until you have cooked all the batter into chaffles.

8. Serve warm and top with sour cream as desired.

Nutrition: Fat 13.4g 17% Carbohydrate 1.3g 0% Sugars 0.6g Protein 46.3g

44. <u>Broccoli Chaffle</u>

Preparation time: 10 minutes

Servings: 4

Difficulty level: Easy

Cooking Time: 15 Minutes

Ingredients:

- Batter

- 4 eggs

- 2 cups grated mozzarella cheese

- 1 cup steamed broccoli, chopped

- Salt and pepper to taste

- 1 clove garlic, minced

- 1 teaspoon chili flakes

- 2 tablespoons almond flour

- 2 teaspoons baking powder

- Other

- 2 tablespoons cooking spray to brush the waffle maker

- ¼ cup mascarpone cheese for serving

Directions:

1. Preheat the waffle maker.

2. Add the eggs, grated mozzarella, chopped broccoli, salt and pepper, minced garlic, chili flakes, almond flour and baking powder to a bowl.

3. Mix with a fork.

4. Brush the heated waffle maker with cooking spray and add a few tablespoons of the batter.

5. Close the lid and cook for about 7 minutes depending on your waffle maker.

6. Serve each chaffle with mascarpone cheese.

Nutrition: Calories 229, fat 15 g, carbs 6 g, sugar 1.1 g, Protein 13.1 g, sodium 194 mg

45. <u>Cocoa Chaffles With Coconut Cream</u>

Preparation time: 9 minutes

Cooking Time: 5 **Ingredients:**

Minutes

Difficulty level: Easy

Servings: 2

- 1 egg

- 1/2 cup mozzarella cheese

- 1 tsp stevia

- 1 tsp vanilla

- 2 tbsps. almond flour

- 1 tbsp. sugar-free chocolate chips

- 2 tbsps. cocoa powder

- TOPPING

- 1 scoop coconut cream

- 1 tbsp. coconut flour

Directions:

1. Mix together chaffle ingredients in a bowl and mix well.

2. Preheat your dash minutes waffle maker. Spray waffle maker with cooking spray.

3. Pour 1/2 batter into the minutes-waffle maker and close the lid.

4. Cook chaffles for about 2-minutesutes and remove from the maker.

5. Make chaffles from the rest of the batter.

6. Serve with a scoop of coconut cream between two chaffles.

7. Drizzle coconut flour on top.

8. Enjoy with afternoon coffee!

Nutrition: Protein: 26% 60 kcal Fat: 65% 152 kcal Carbohydrates: 21 kcal

46. <u>Keto Pizza Chaffle</u>

Preparation time: 9 minutes

Difficulty level: Easy

Cooking Time: 15 Minutes

Servings: 2

Ingredients:

- Pizza Filing: 1/3 cups pepperoni slices

- 1 tbsp marinara sauce

- ½ cup shredded mozzarella cheese

- 1 onion (finely chopped)

- 1 small green bell pepper (finely chopped)

- Chaffle: 1 egg (beaten)

- A pinch of Italian seasoning

- A pinch of salt

- ½ cup mozzarella cheese ¼ tsp baking powder

- ½ tsp dried basil A pinch of garlic powder

- 1 tbsp + 1 tsp almond flour

Directions:

1. Preheat the oven to 400°F and line a baking sheet with parchment paper.

2. Plug the waffle maker and preheat it. Spray it with a nonstick spray.

3. For the chaffle: In a mixing bowl, combine the baking powder, almond flour, garlic powder, Italian seasoning, basil, mozzarella cheese and salt. Add the egg and mix until the ingredients are well combined.

4. Fill the waffle maker with appropriate amount of the batter and spread the batter to the edges of the waffle maker to cover all the holes on the waffle maker.

5. Close the lid of the waffle maker and cook for about minutes or according to waffle maker's settings.

6. After the baking cycle, remove the chaffle from waffle maker with a silicone or plastic utensil.

7. Repeat step 4 to 6 until you have cooked all the batter into chaffles.

8. Top each of the chaffles with the marinara sauce, sprinkle the finely chopped onions and pepper over the chaffles.

9. Top with shredded mozzarella cheese and layer the pepperoni slices on the cheese topping.

10. Gently place the chaffles on the lined baking sheet. Place the baking sheet in the oven and bake for about 5 minutes. Afterwards, broil for about 1 minute.

11. Remove the pizza chaffles from the oven and let them cook for a few minutes.

12. Serve warm and enjoy.

Nutrition: Fat 23.2g 30% Carbohydrate 14.9g 5% Sugars 6.8g Protein 16.8g

47. <u>Double Cheese Chaffles With Mayonnaise</u> <u>Dip</u>

Preparation time: 9 minutes

Difficulty level: Easy

Cooking Time: 8 Minutes

Servings: 2

Ingredients:

- Chaffles

- ½ cup mozzarella cheese, shredded

- 1 tablespoon Parmesan cheese, shredded

- 1 organic egg

- ¾ teaspoon coconut flour

- ¼ teaspoon organic baking powder

- 1/8 teaspoon Italian seasoning

- Pinch of salt

- Dip

- ¼ cup mayonnaise

- Pinch of garlic powder

- Pinch of ground black pepper

Directions:

1. Preheat a mini waffle iron and then grease it.

2. For chaffles: In a medium bowl, put all ingredients and with a fork, mix until well combined. Place half of the mixture into preheated waffle iron and cook for about 3–4 minutes.

3. Repeat with the remaining mixture.

4. Meanwhile, for dip: in a bowl, mix together the cream and stevia.

5. Serve warm chaffles alongside the dip.

Nutrition: Calories 248 Net Carbs 1.2 g Total Fat 24.3 g Saturated Fat 4.9 g Cholesterol 98 mg Sodium 374 mg Total Carbs 1.g Fiber 0.4 g Sugar 0.2 g Protein 5.9 g

48. <u>Chaffles With Chocolate Balls</u>

Preparation time: 9 minutes

Difficulty level: Easy

Servings: 2

Cooking Time: 5 Minutes

Ingredients:

- 1/4 cup heavy cream

- ½ cup unsweetened cocoa powder

- 1/4 cup coconut meat

- CHAFFLE Ingredients:

- 1 egg

- ½ cup mozzarella cheese

Directions:

1. Make 2 chaffles with chaffle ingredients.

2. Meanwhile, mix together all ingredients in a mixing bowl.

3. Make two balls from the mixture and freeze in the freezer for about 2 hours until set.

4. Serve with keto chaffles and enjoy!

Nutrition: Protein: 18% 46 kcal Fat: 78% 196 kcal Carbohydrates: 4% 10 kcal

CHAPTER 13:

CHAFFLE MEAT RECIPES

49. Classic Ground Pork Chaffle

Preparation time: 10 minutes

Difficulty level: Easy

Cooking Time: 15 Minutes **Servings:** 2

Ingredients:

- ½ pound ground pork

- 3 eggs

- ½ cup grated mozzarella cheese

- Salt and pepper to taste

- 1 clove garlic, minced

- 1 teaspoon dried oregano

- Other

- 2 tablespoons butter to brush the waffle maker

- 2 tablespoons freshly chopped parsley for garnish

Directions:

1. Preheat the waffle maker.

2. Add the ground pork, eggs, mozzarella cheese, salt and pepper, minced garlic and dried oregano to a bowl. Mix until combined.

3. Brush the heated waffle maker with butter and add a few tablespoons of the batter.

4. Close the lid and cook for about 7–8 minutes depending on your waffle maker. Serve with freshly chopped parsley.

Nutrition: Calories 192, fat 11.g, carbs 1 g, sugar 0.3 g, Protein 20.2 g, sodium 142 mg

50. <u>Turkey Chaffle Sandwich</u>

Preparation time: 10 minutes

Difficulty level: Easy

Cooking Time: 15 Minutes **Servings:** 2

Ingredients:

- Batter

- 4 eggs

- ¼ cup cream cheese

- 1 cup grated mozzarella cheese

- Salt and pepper to taste

- 1 teaspoon dried dill

- ½ teaspoon onion powder

- ½ teaspoon garlic powder

- Juicy chicken

- 2 tablespoons butter

- 1 pound chicken breast

- Salt and pepper to taste

- 1 teaspoon dried dill

- 2 tablespoons heavy cream

- Other

- 2 tablespoons butter to brush the waffle maker

- 4 lettuce leaves to garnish the sandwich

- 4 tomato slices to garnish the sandwich

Directions:

1. Preheat the waffle maker.

2. Add the eggs, cream cheese, mozzarella cheese, salt and pepper, dried dill, onion powder and garlic powder to a bowl.

3. Mix everything with a fork just until batter forms.

4. Brush the heated waffle maker with butter and add a few tablespoons of the batter. Close the lid and cook for about 7 minutes depending on your waffle maker.

5. Meanwhile, heat some butter in a nonstick pan.

6. Season the chicken with salt and pepper and sprinkle with dried dill. Pour the heavy cream on top.

7. Cook the chicken slices for about 10 minutes or until golden brown.

8. Cut each chaffle in half.

9. On one half add a lettuce leaf, tomato slice, and chicken slice. Cover with the other chaffle half to make a sandwich. Serve and enjoy.

Nutrition: Calories 381, fat 26.3 g, carbs 2.5 g, sugar 1 g, Protein 32.9 g, sodium 278 mg

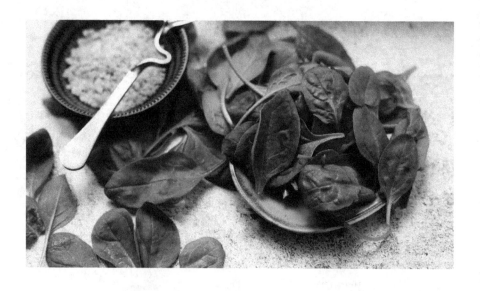

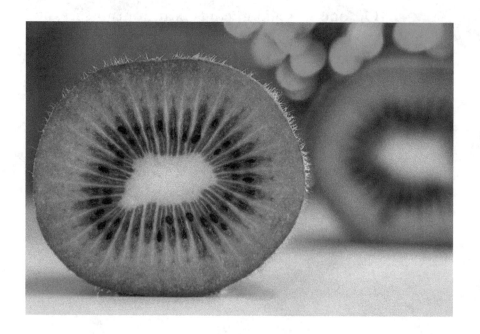

CONCLUSION

In the low-carb world, the word 'CHAFFLE' appeared and took the social media by storm. The waffle maker became the need of every keto kitchen and individuals following ketogenic diet found their new love. This new addition in the keto diet is not only healthy but the possibilities to experiment with new recipes are countless.

Furthermore, it has also made it easy for keto followers to follow their diet and controlling their cravings for flour based foods. In simple words, chaffles are the low-carb waffles – they are called chaffle because cheese is used as their base ingredient. Cheese and waffle by combining these words you will get the delicious chaffles.

Another benefit that we offer? We explain routines that you can do for yourself to make this diet last longer for you and to benefit your body better as a result. Routines are very important and can be a big help to your body but also your spirit and your mind.

This will help you utilize the diet better, and you will be able to improve with it as well as have it become easier for you to handle. You want to stay healthy and make sure that your body is able to do what it needs to.

As with anything, we have put a strong emphasis on the fact that if anything feels wrong or unnatural, you will need to see a doctor to make sure that you are safe and that your body can handle this diet. Use the knowledge in this book to have amazing recipes and learn how to prepare amazing meals for you.

How to Clean and Maintain the Waffle Maker

Make sure that it is not hot before you clean the waffle or chaffle maker. But clean it as soon as it is cool enough.

1. Use a damp cloth or paper towel for wiping away the crumbs.
2. Soak up the excess oil drips on your grid plates.
3. Wipe the exterior with the damp cloth or paper towel.
4. Pour a few drops of cooking oil on the batter to remove the stubborn batter drips. Wipe it away after this.
5. You can wash the cooking plates in soapy warm water. Rinse them clean.

6. Ensure that the waffle maker is completely dry before storing it.

Waffle Maker Maintenance Tips

Remember these simple tips and your waffle maker will serve you for a long time.

- Instruction manual should be well read before you use it for the first time.
- Only a light cooking oil coating is required for nonstick waffle makers.
- Grease the grid with only a little amount of oil if you see the waffles sticking.
- Never use metal or sharp tools to scrape off the batter or to remove the cooked waffles. You may end up scratching the surface and damaging it.
- Do not submerge your electric waffle maker in water.

Chaffles can be frozen and processed, so a large proportion can be made and stored for quick and extremely fast meals. If you don't have a waffle maker, just cook the mixture like a pancake in a frying pan, or even cooler, in a fryer-pan. They won't get all the fluffy sides to achieve like you're using a waffle maker, but they're definitely going to taste great.

Depending on which cheese you choose, the carbs and net calorie number can shift a little bit. However, in general, whether you use real, whole milk cheese, chaffles are completely carb-free.

For up to a month, chaffles will be frozen. However, defrosting them absorbs plenty of moist, which makes it difficult to get their crisp again. Chaffles are rich in fat and moderate in protein and low in carb. Chaffle is a very well established and popular technique to hold people on board.

And the chaffles are more durable and better than most forms of keto bread. "What a high-carb diet you may be desirous of. A nonstick waffle maker is something that makes life easier, and it's a trade-off that's happy to embrace for our wellbeing.

CPSIA information can be obtained
at www.ICGtesting.com
Printed in the USA
BVHW011623100521
606949BV00002B/150

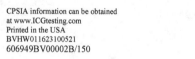

9 781802 671971